Linda Ljucovic, part owner of Balance Point Health Centre in Oakville, graduated from Mc-Master University in 1992 with a BA in Labour Studies and went on to complete her Human Resources Certification in 1994. Throughout her career in Human Resources, specifically learning and development and organizational development, she focused on teaching the skills for effective goal setting, coaching and leadership. Learning and teaching have always been a passion of Linda's.

Linda obtained her Classic Hatha Yoga certification in 2001 from the Hatha/Raja Yoga Studies school in Toronto where she learned from the talented Marie Paulyn, founder of Federation of Ontario's Yoga Teachers (FOYT). Linda has taught on and off on a part time basis in corporate and private settings.

Through her own personal health challenges and those of her children, she has become passionate about the study of nutrition and its effect on the mind and body. Linda went on to complete her study at the Canadian School of Natural Nutrition in 2012 and is now a Registered Holistic Nutritionist (RHN). She is motivated by helping others learn about how the food we eat impacts every aspect of our lives and that even simple and gradual changes can lead to improved health and a renewed passion for life.

Lisa Van Meeteren has over 15 years of experience working as a freelance copywriter, and has worked for clients such as Visa and Hallmark and everything in between. Graduating from Ryerson's Radio and Television arts she specialized in Media Copywriting, and then went on to complete the post graduate Copywriting program at Humber College.

She met Linda when she was struggling with a myriad of hormone related health issues including PMS and was seeking a way to change for the better. While Lisa cooks a little, she likes to eat a lot and like many of us can make poor food choices. Educating herself about nutrition and the impact it can have on our health has been enlightening to Lisa and she looks forward to implementing the eating principles that she has learned while writing this book. She has completed a novel, several plays and is always writing something. This is her first cookbook.

Table of Contents

This book is more than just a cookbook! It is a health guide and cookbook wrapped into one neat little package designed to help you conquer your PMS.

This book will:

- Help you learn why you have PMS.
- Teach you to take control by making healthier food choices.
- Provide up to date nutritional information and health supportive recipes made from real ingredients.
- Provide you with a menu plan aimed at reducing PMS.

All recipes are simple and easy and were created with the following PMS guidelines for nutrition in mind.

PMS Nutritional Guidelines

- Limit dairy
- Eat low glycemic foods and keep sugar, caffeine and alcohol to a minimum!
- Ban if you can – but at the very least, reduce 'white foods' that have very little nutritive value – refined sugar and white flour products that rob your body of nutrition
- Avoid high fat animal products (beef, pork, lamb) as they have been found to increase symptoms and pain.
- Avoid wheat products that can contribute to inflammation in your body
- Increase fibre, A, B, and E vitamins, long chain fatty acids, calcium, magnesium and zinc.
- Choose hormone-free eggs, dairy and meat.
- Choose pure filtered water and avoid drinking water from plastic bottles.

Overall, focus on high fibre, healthy lean protein and healthy fats and limit refined sugar.

So let's get started!
It's time to begin feeling like yourself
again no matter what time of the month it is!

There are three little letters in the alphabet that when put together can become a powerful enemy in a woman's life. P-M-S. That's right, we're talking about PMS; a very real, very frustrating syndrome that can take a huge physical and emotional toll on you, making your life and the lives of those around you downright miserable. You may wonder why you often turn into someone you're not (overly emotional, a craving lunatic, highly temperamental), or why you simply feel like you're out of control. The good news is, once you understand the causes of PMS, you are more motivated to make the changes that are necessary for a more hormonally balanced cycle. This section will provide recipes and information on how you can take back control and get some relief from premenstrual symptoms through nutrition.

Why me?

Experts say that 90 percent of all women between the ages of 20 and 50 experience some degree of PMS, so you're not alone! Symptoms such as headaches, acne, food cravings, bloating, constipation or diarrhea and mood swings can last anywhere from 2 days to as long as 2 weeks*; no wonder so many of us are cranky! The shift in our hormones, specifically the ratios of estrogen to progesterone during the menstrual cycle is thought to be the major cause of PMS but there are many other contributing factors. Poor nutrition as well as unstable blood sugar levels aggravate PMS. PMS may also be linked to food allergies, changes in carbohydrate metabolism, hypoglycemia, mineral and/or vitamin deficiencies, difficulty absorbing and utilizing fatty acids and a malfunction in the brain's mood regulator...phew! That's some list! So where to begin? Start where you have complete control - the food that you eat! It's easy to make small tweaks to see if it makes a difference for you. If you don't see results after trying the suggestions in this book for at least 3 months, you may want to consider seeing a Naturopath or Nutritionist to explore the possibility of food allergies or one of the other causes mentioned above.

What causes the imbalances in the first place?

Does constantly running, looking at the clock, pumping yourself full of caffeine and sugar to make it through the day sound familiar? This daily routine that many of us follow makes us feel as though we are running on empty and our busy stressed out lives begin to create imbalances in our endocrine systems:

- You may experience low levels of serotonin, the chemical in your brain that makes you feel happy.
- You may have low levels of vitamins D and B, and minerals such as magnesium.
- A stressed out liver may lead to troubles processing estrogens which can lead to an excess of these hormones in the body and prostaglandin imbalance.

All these factors may contribute to PMS.

Food Facts...

"Food plays a huge role in how we function on a daily basis both on a physical level and emotional level. Our food acts as the building blocks for all aspects of us - hair, skin, lungs, liver, brain ... and yes even our moods. There is significant truth in the quote 'One man's food is another man's poison.' Food sensitivity testing is a wonderful tool to pinpoint individual food intolerances. When my patients are able to eliminate their specific aggravating foods they see improvement in both their physical and emotional health concerns. This is even the case for those struggling with mood changes and PMS. PMS doesn't have to be something we suffer through every month."

Dr. Jennifer Kaster, ND
Balance Point Health Centre, Oakville, ON

Help me!! What can I do?

You can help put back the missing links in your system by:

- following a healthy diet chock full of nutrition
- exercising regularly
- adding calming activities to your routine such as yoga or meditation

However, the most important thing for right now is to get your blood sugar levels under control. The cravings for sugar and high fat foods come from dysglycemia, a term that basically means your blood sugar is as dysfunctional as the *Desperate Housewives of Orange County*. If your blood sugar levels are constantly going up and down then your moods will follow. Make sure your meals and snacks are balanced with some protein and slow releasing carbohydrates to help keep your blood sugar stable. Even better, remove those things robbing your system of nutrients and happiness in the first place, like caffeine, alcohol and sugar and you will be well on your way to winning the war against PMS. You may also want to increase your intake of tryptophan or 5 HTP which many of the recipes in this book naturally do.

Another way to help PMS is by removing certain foods that can do more harm than good during this time such as dairy. Research shows that women who cut dairy from their diets for ten days prior to their periods do notice a significant decrease in their PMS symptoms. To make it easier for you, most of the recipes in this section are dairy free and have good levels of calcium!

It can be overwhelming to implement so many changes at once; so start with a small change. If you're not exercising, simply start walking. If you're eating too much refined sugar, replace a sweet with one of the delectable treat recipes in this book. Take it slow and implement a few recipes in the book right before you typically experience PMS and take notice of how you feel.

Once you start to feel better you will be encouraged to follow the other suggestions. And don't worry, this isn't a super strict 'avoid every grain and sugar' type of recipe book. (Not that there's anything wrong with that … but we wanted to make this realistic and when we are PMS'ing – often the best plans get thrown out the window in exchange for a chocolate brownie). Luckily, there are plenty of healthy recipes in this book to indulge your sweet tooth, including brownies. Luckier yet, they are loaded with only natural sugars and ingredients that won't derail your efforts to feel better and get healthy. This plan is about getting more nutrition – it is not about deprivation or eating less.

Each recipe is designed to supply your body with the nutrients that women with PMS tend to be deficient in to reduce symptoms. Since we are all biochemically different, some will work better for you than others, just pay attention to your symptoms and the changes in your body along the way and you will be able to piece together the changes you need to make to keep your PMS under control.

So let's get started. Remember to give yourself permission to slow down during the weeks leading up to your period. Find at least 30 minutes a day to nurture yourself, without the guilt. Read a book, go to yoga, go on a walk with a neighbour and/or friend, meditate, breathe deeply for 5 minutes, and eat your food slowly and mindfully. We know it is easier said than done. In the long run these small nurturing acts for yourself will spill over into other areas of your life, and you will be enjoying some delicious food in the process … sounds like a win-win to us!

Vitamin A – according to the Weston Price Foundation, vitamin A has proven beneficial in reducing some PMS symptoms. Be sure to use a natural source of this nutrient, such as cod liver oil, as synthetic versions can be toxic.

Pantothenic acid – always desirable for treating stress.

Vitamin E – good for sore breasts and for regulating hormonal levels, irritability and depression .

Calcium and magnesium – pivotal in reducing stress, as well as encouraging proper muscle function; important in eradicating painful cramping and nervous tension.

Long-chain fatty acids – prompts the release of anti-inflammatory substances known as prostaglandins; gamma-linoleic acid or GLA, has been shown to be of special value in resolving PMS and other ailments. It is found in evening primrose oil, borage oil or black currant oil.

Natural sources of PMS Nutritional Powerhouses

Vitamin A	Cod liver oil, liver (avoid due to toxins), butter, egg yolks
Vitamin D	Oily fish, lard, cod liver oil
Vitamin B6	Brown rice, liver, beef, whole wheat, rye, lentils, alfalfa, tuna, peas, bananas, cashews, turkey, oats, blackstrap molasses, cabbage
Pantothenic Acid	Brewer's yeast, brown rice, sunflower seeds, corn, lentils, whole wheat, rye
Vitamin E	Fresh wheat germ, wheat germ oil, whole wheat, raw nuts, olive oil, peanuts, broccoli, pecans
Calcium	Raw milk and raw milk cheeses, bone broths, sesame seeds, kelp, sardines, almonds, brazil nuts, blackstrap molasses, watercress, dark green leafy vegetables, salmon, broccoli
Magnesium	Kelp, beef, blackstrap molasses, sunflower seeds, all nuts, oats, brown rice, dark green leafy vegetables, corn, bananas, tuna
Fatty Acids	Cod liver oil, salmon, sardines, mackerel, egg yolks and borage, black currant or evening primrose oil

See your Doctor or Naturopath when...

- Your symptoms become so strong that they interfere with your daily life
- You show signs of depression that occur regularly during your menstrual cycle, including food cravings, crying, insomnia, emotional withdrawal and mood swings.

Most things that are good for us are good in moderation. The moment we have too much of something even if it is considered "healthy" our bodies aren't sure what to do with it. This is true for the most part with wheat products. Wheat is everywhere. In addition to the breads, crackers, baked goods, cereals and pastas that you consume, wheat is also added to many other products you wouldn't even suspect like soup, sauces, dressings, and most processed and packaged food.

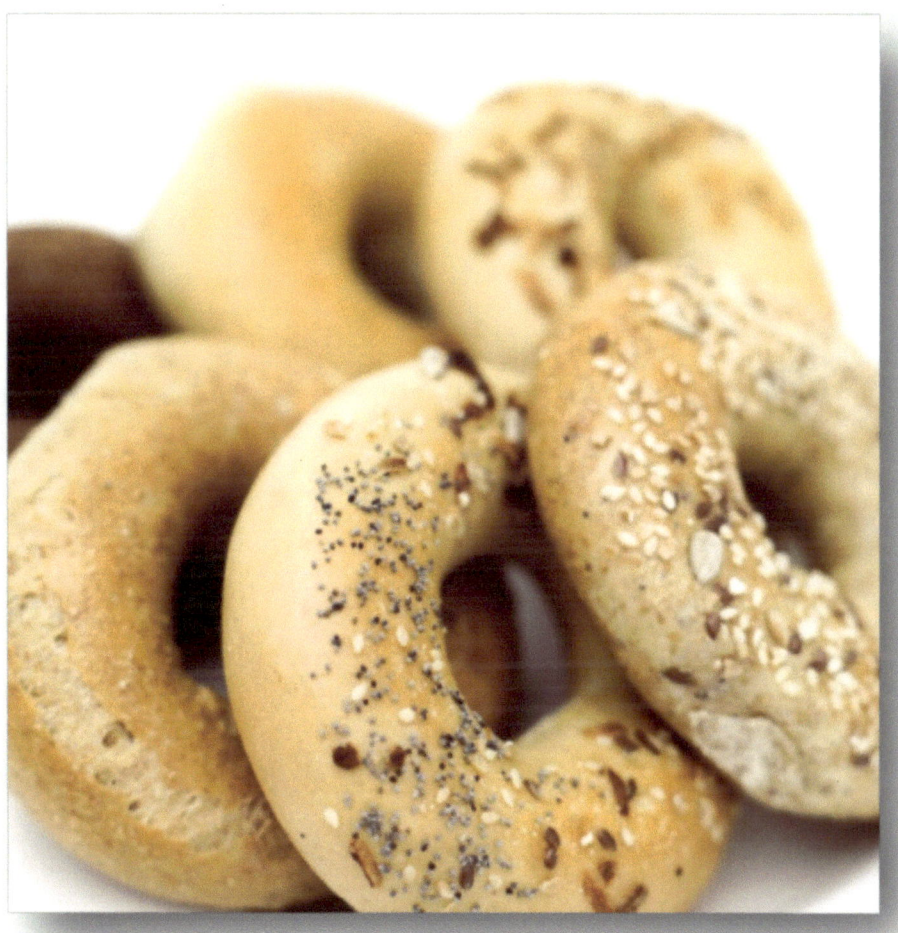

Though wheat can be a healthy grain, eating too much of it can cause issues, leading to food intolerances and allergies. And like we just said, too much of a good thing is too much … which could explain why many have become intolerant to this grain in recent years. Our bodies are reacting to its excessive intake with an allergenic and immune response.

Many argue that the wheat that our parents ate isn't the wheat of today. Modern day wheat has at least twenty times more gluten then the wheat of the past! No wonder our bodies can't tolerate it anymore. Wheat has been found to cause mood imbalances and bloating in some people, so if you suffer from those symptoms, you might want to consider eliminating this grain for a period of time to see if it helps. Many an ache, pain, and mood swing has been cured by putting down the bagels and going wheat free. Try substituting other grains wherever possible and if you think you have issues with wheat you may want to try cutting it out altogether to see how you feel.

Your nutritionist or naturopath may be able to provide you some guidance on going wheat free.

These muffins taste delicious but because they are grain free, they may look different than what you're used to. Most muffins that you buy at your local coffee shop or store contain processed ingredients and unhealthy fats that give them a nice fluffy texture and shiny gleam. Unfortunately, that shiny gleam comes from sugar, and that fluffiness, from processed flour. Our muffins will keep you going much longer and are loaded with nutrition like B vitamins, fibre and healthy fats. This muffin makes a nice afternoon snack and won't lead to fluctuations in your blood sugar levels. So go ahead and indulge in a muffin that won't give you a muffin top!

Ingredients

- ½ cup coconut flour
- ¼ tsp salt
- ½ tsp baking powder
- 6 hormone free eggs
- 4 tbsp coconut oil
- ¼ cup honey (or agave or sweetener of choice)
- 2 small ripe bananas, mashed
- ½ cup chopped walnuts and/or dark chocolate chips

Directions

Preheat oven to 350°F. Combine flour, salt, baking powder and walnuts in one bowl. Mix eggs, melted coconut oil, honey and mashed banana in another bowl. Mix dry ingredients with wet ingredients until combined. Spoon into paper lined muffin tins – about ¾ full. Bake at 350°F for 25 minutes or until done.

RECIPE TIP

Coconut flour is very dry! You will notice that it absorbs the liquid quickly. However, coconut has many healing qualities and has also been found to increase metabolism and encourage weight loss. Coconut flour is a good alternative to grain flours which many people are becoming intolerant to.

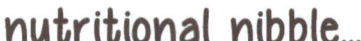

nutritional nibble...

Bananas are high in potassium, while walnuts are high in Omega 3's – the good fats that help keep our mood balanced. Essential fatty acids help our body function better emotionally and physically and help us to metabolize our food more effectively. Don't worry about good fat making you fat - just like chocolate, not all fats are created equal.

Okay, so you're going to crave carbs this time of the month so don't deny those cravings. Instead, why not trade... why not trade in your favourite sugar and refined carbohydrate laden muffin with one that is filled with mood boosting essential fatty acids (EFA's) from energy boosting whole oats? It will satisfy your craving without sending your blood sugar and mood on a roller coaster ride. Oh and we've also thrown in some chocolate for an extra burst of happiness. You're welcome!

Ingredients

- 1 ¼ cup oats (optional: grind oats)
- ½ cup brown rice flour, spelt flour or whole wheat flour
- ⅓ cup cocoa powder
- ¼ cup ground flaxseed
- ½ tsp baking soda
- sprinkle of sea salt
- 1 tsp baking powder
- 2 eggs, beaten (or 2 tbsp of ground flax seeds mixed into 6 tbsp water)
- ¼ cup plain yogurt or almond milk
- 2 medium, ripe bananas, mashed
- ¼ cup molasses, agave syrup or coconut sugar
- 5 tbsp grapeseed oil or melted coconut oil
- ¼ cup walnuts and/or dark chocolate chips

Directions

Preheat oven to 375°F. In a large bowl, whisk together oats, flour, cocoa powder, flaxseed, baking soda, sea salt and baking powder. In a separate bowl, combine eggs, yogurt, bananas, syrup and oil. Add flour mixture and fold together with walnuts. Divide batter into 12 paper-lined muffin cups. Bake for 20 – 22 minutes or until tops spring back when lightly touched. Cool on wire rack or eat when warm.

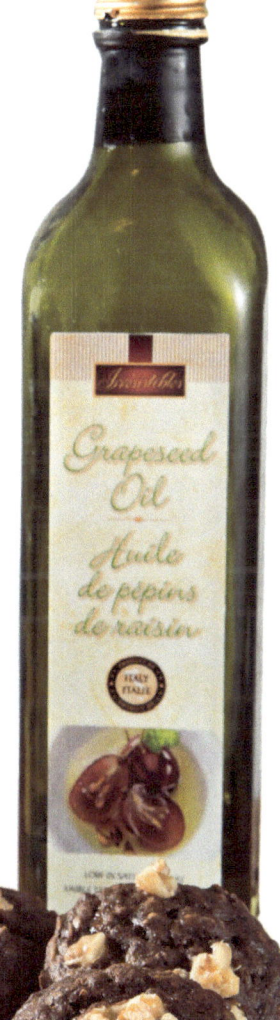

Did you know?

Grapeseed oil does not break down at high temperatures like olive oil, so is a great oil to use for baking and stir fries. The antioxidants in grapeseed oil are also fifty times higher than those found in vitamin C: you won't find that in regular vegetable oil (an oil known to break down after being heated). Plus as an extra bonus, it contains linoleic acid, an essential fatty acid important to the health of our skin. Use it as a moisturizer to make your skin soft and reduce the unwanted signs of aging. (Wow! Maybe they sell it in giant Costco tubs so we can bathe in it!)

If your first thought when you hear GI is Joe then you might be in trouble...

If you want to fight off mood swings, cravings and weight gain (all things too common in PMS) focus on foods with a low glycemic index (GI) rating. Here's a little background on the Glycemic Index:

Low-GI carbs take much longer to digest, providing the body with a slow, steady supply of energy. The 'GI' rating of a food refers to how quickly the food converts to sugar in our bodies. High fibre foods and whole foods have lower glycemic index ratings for example than lower fibre, highly processed foods. Refined carbs, like white rice or juice have a high GI rating as they are quickly broken down by the body causing rapid fluctuations in blood glucose levels, which as we now know can aggravate PMS (among other things!).

You can lower the GI rating of foods by combining low GI foods with high GI foods. For example, adding walnuts to your oatmeal will lower the GI rating of your meal.

Please keep in mind that a little common sense goes a long way when using the GI index. There are foods such as certain candy bars that contain nuts that have a lower GI mainly because the fat and protein counteracts the sugar but obviously a chocolate bar shouldn't be your go to when you're trying to eat more healthfully. The bottom line for good blood sugar balance and better overall health, as previously mentioned, is to always combine a protein with a complex carb. Choose whole grains over refined grains and try to opt for more root and leafy vegetables to make up the carb portion of your diet. Quality is more important than quantity.

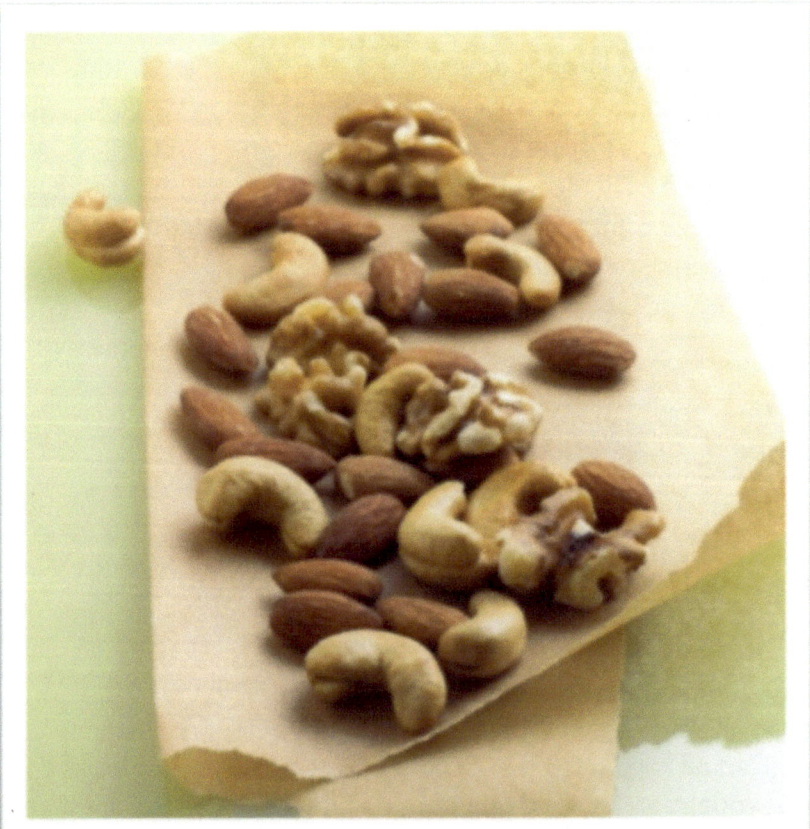

High GI Foods

White bread, baked potato, instant rice, cooked carrots, corn flakes, white rice products, wheat, puffed cereal, sweetened cereals, most pasta, maltose, glucose, raisins, honey, refined sugar, watermelon, dried apricots, pineapples, ripe bananas.

Low GI Foods

Whole oats, wild rice, quinoa, whole spelt, sweet potatoes, green beans, peas, nuts, seeds, black beans, kidney beans, butter beans, tomatoes, artichokes, asparagus, pears, peaches, apples, yogurt with fruit, stevia.

Ingredients

- ⅓ cup whole oats (wheat free version)
- 1 tsp lecithin
- 2 tbsp wheat germ (go B6 go!)
- 1 tbsp ground flax seeds or chia seeds
- 1 tbsp nutritional yeast
- 3 dried, chopped apricots or berries
- splash of unsweetened almond milk
- maple syrup or stevia to taste

Directions

Cook oats in ⅔ cups of pure water for 15 minutes. Sprinkle all other ingredients on oatmeal and enjoy! If you are missing any of the ingredients listed above, just use what you have, as long as you include a healthy fat and additional protein.

Did you know?

Lecithin is a lipid or fat that is important to the entire body, ensuring proper brain and nerve function. Basically, it makes up the protective sheath of the brain and nervous systems. Lecithin comes from soybean, sprouts and eggs. It contains choline (B vitamin), inositol, and linoleic acid (an omega-6 fatty acid). So what does this mean to you? Healthy nervous system function improves the body's ability to counter stress. Less stress = more happiness! And happiness is a welcome benefit during PMS.

FUN FACT

Mornings can be hectic… tempting most of us to use quick cooking oats instead of the slow cooking ones. The problem with that is the faster the cereal cooks the higher its rating on the GI. How to overcome this without a time machine? Use a crock pot. Place 1 cup of oatmeal with 2 cups of water in the crock pot with a little sea salt and then turn on low overnight. You can add your almond milk and toppings in the morning and voila, instant breakfast that won't be 'instant' in quality.

nutritional nibble…

Nutritional Yeast is commonly used by vegetarians and vegans for its nutty, cheese-like flavor. It is loaded with vitamins and minerals, is high in fibre, low in salt, high in B Vitamins (especially B12), and is naturally low in fat. Try it on popcorn!

Note: Some people find they are sensitive to nutritional yeast so like with any new food, introduce it slowly into your diet and watch for any adverse reactions like a scratchy throat, changes in your BMs (yes we said it), rashes, etc.

Many of us who are trying to increase our protein start our day with a healthy smoothie. But there are some mornings where you crave something a little more comforting. That doesn't mean you need to derail your efforts to eat healthy. These delicious, high protein pancakes are low on the glycemic index, high in fibre and full of healthy fats to fill you up so you won't even think about lunch…until, well, lunch. Plus they're delicious and gluten free!

Ingredients

- 1 tbsp vanilla extract
- 1 ½ cups blanched almond flour
- ¼ tsp baking soda
- 3 eggs
- sprinkle of stevia
- ¼ tsp celtic sea salt
- grapeseed oil , for cooking
- 1 tbsp water

Directions

In a large bowl whisk together eggs, water, vanilla and stevia. Add almond flour, salt and baking soda and mix until thoroughly combined. Heat grapeseed oil on skillet over medium low to medium heat. Scoop one heaping tablespoon of batter at a time onto the skillet. Pancakes will form little bubbles. When bubbles open, flip pancakes over and cook the other side. Remove from heat to a plate. Repeat process with remaining batter; add more oil to skillet as needed. Top with 2 tablespoons of organic Greek yogurt, berries of choice and a sprinkle of stevia.

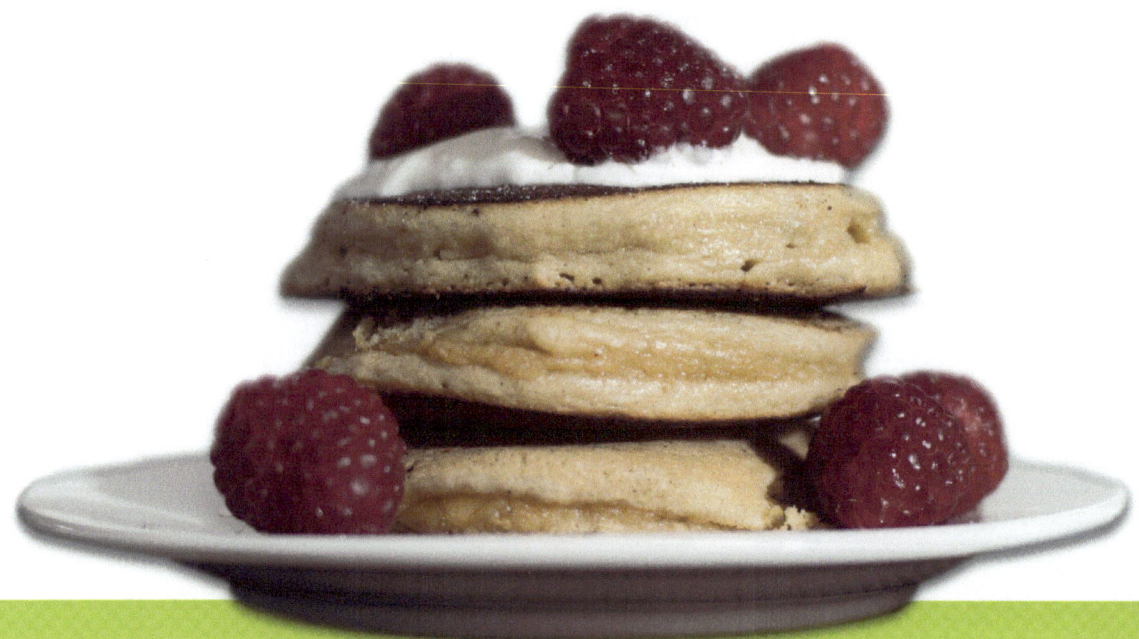

nutritional nibble...

Almonds are low on the glycemic scale, which again means that they help reduce the rise in sugar and insulin levels after meals. They are also high in fibre and healthy fats, two key ingredients for reducing PMS symptoms over the long term.

Did you Know?

Primrose oil has been found to reduce the symptoms of PMS if taken during the last half of your cycle. Talk to your nutritionist or Naturopath to see if this is the right option for you.

Chocolate Raspberry Delight Smoothie : Serves 1

Who doesn't love the combination of chocolate and raspberries together? This smoothie rivals any four star dessert in taste, while helping to lift your mood and shrink your waistline. Bottoms up!

Ingredients

- 1 scoop of vanilla whey protein powder
- 1 cup frozen raspberries
- 4 – 5 raw cacao beans or 1 tbsp raw cacao
- ½ banana
- 1 tbsp chia seeds
- 1 tbsp lecithin granules
- ½ cup of almond milk
- ½ – 1 cup water

Directions

Blend all ingredients together using a food processor or blender. Enjoy!

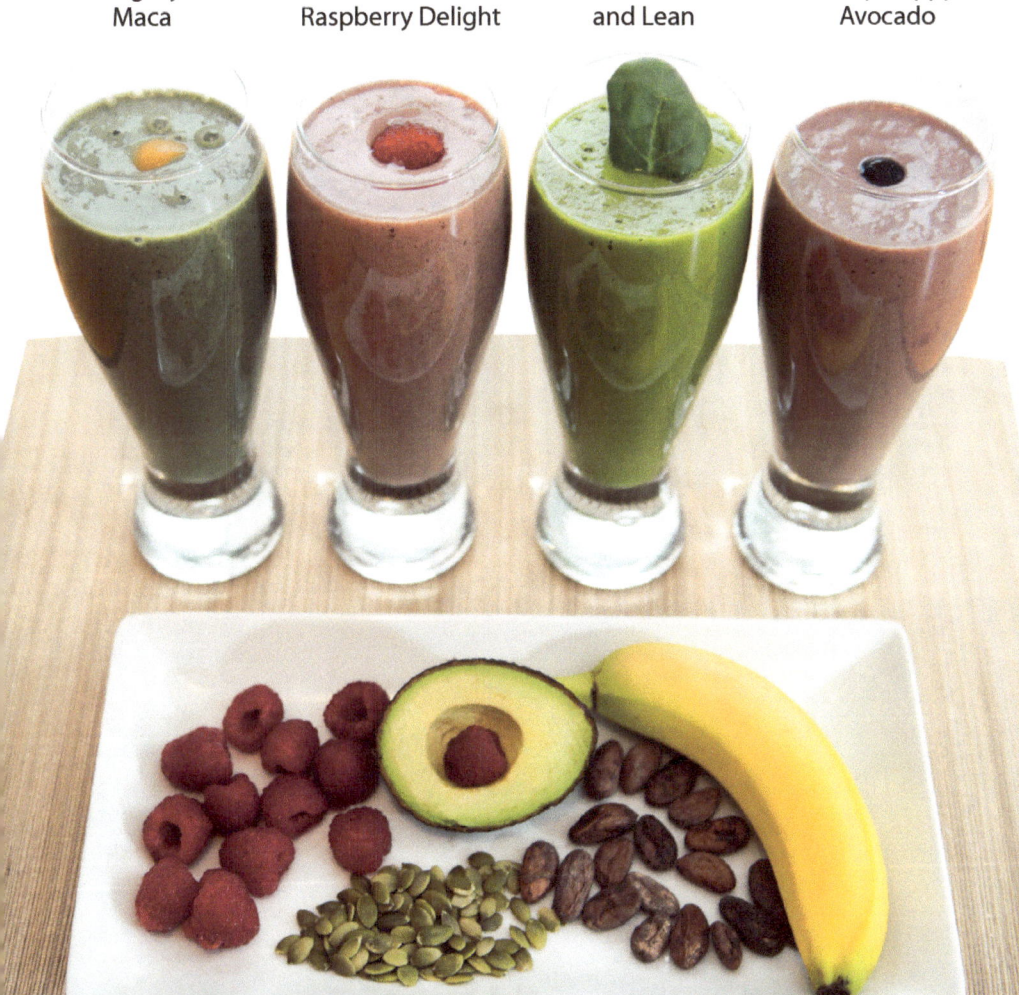

Mighty
Maca

Chocolate
Raspberry Delight

Be Green
and Lean

Berry Happy
Avocado

nutritional nibble...

Hooray for whey! Whey protein powder is a high quality form of protein that boosts the body's store of an important amino acid called glutathione. Glutathione is an antioxidant that mops up free radicals and is involved in the detoxification of carcinogens. The white blood cells and the liver both use glutathione to detoxify poisons in the body. Glutathione needs to be manufactured in the body, and one of the best building blocks is whey protein powder. During PMS, any support you can provide to your liver will help it to focus on all of its functions, like processing hormones and managing your PMS.

Berry Happy Avocado Shake: Serves 1

Okay move over frosted cereal! This protein shake is easy and portable, making it a perfect meal to take on the run. High in nutrients and delicious, it has healthy fats to keep you satisfied and happy, and protein to keep your blood sugar and your mood stable. Say good-bye sugary grains and hello to happiness and stability! Cheers!

Ingredients

- 1 serving protein powder – vanilla (whey isolate or vegan)
- ¼ cup frozen berries
- 1 tsp cacao powder
- ¼ avocado
- ½ tbsp ground pumpkin seeds
- 1 tbsp flax oil
- 1 tbsp lecithin granules
- water (fill glass you will be drinking from ¾ full)

Directions

Blend protein powder, berries, cacao powder, avocado, pumpkin seeds and chia seeds. (Vita Mix works excellently but any blender should work.)

nutritional nibble…

Pumpkin seeds are an excellent source of B vitamins such as:
- thiamin
- riboflavin
- niacin
- pantothenic acid
- vitamin B-6 (pyridoxine)
- and folates.

Niacin helps reduce LDL – cholesterol levels in the blood which is important for a healthy heart.

Along with glutamate, it enhances GABA activity inside the brain, which helps reduce anxiety… something that couldcome in handy during those PMS days.

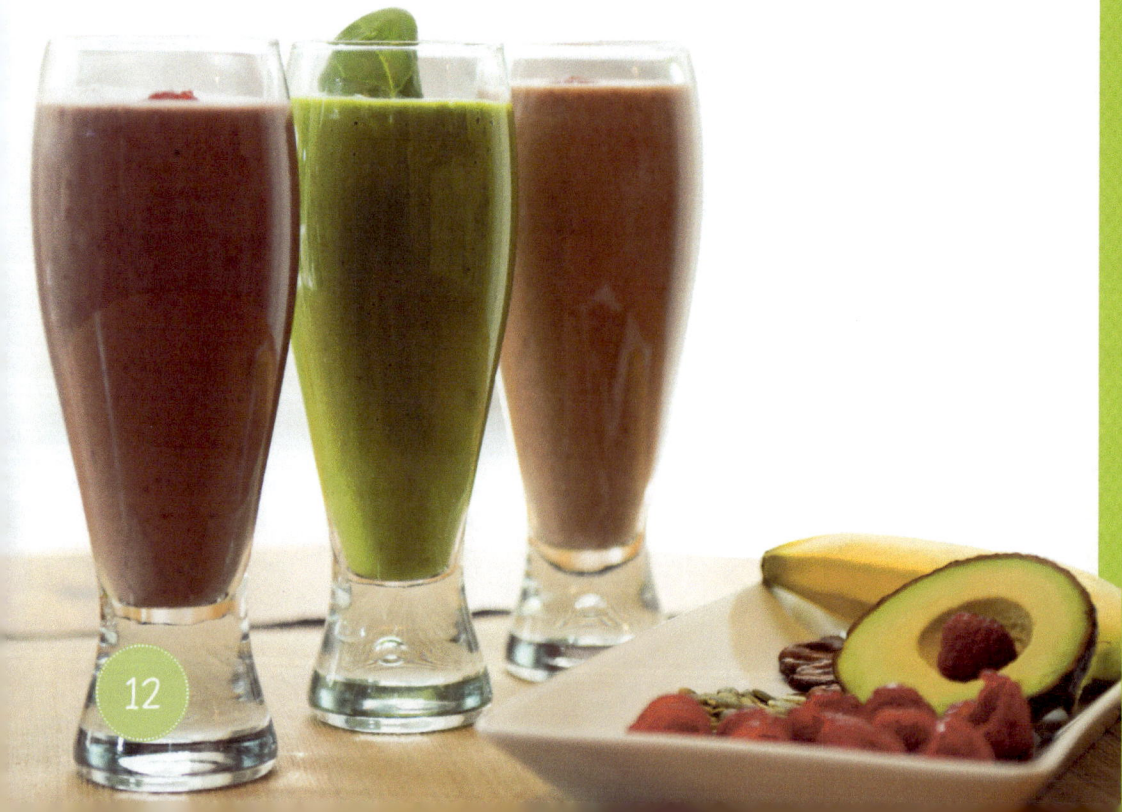

Sorry Kermit and those of you who complain it's not easy to be green…now it is. Sneak in an extra serving of greens for an added health boost in this smoothie. You won't notice the greens taste but you will notice the energy they provide to keep you going all morning long. If you aren't a breakfast eater or are pressed for time in the morning then this is a great option.

Ingredients

- 1 – 2 cups water (depending on how thick you like it)
- ½ – 1 cup frozen peaches
- ¼ avocado
- 1 tbsp Udo's Oil or Flax Oil
- 1 tbsp chia seeds
- 1 scoop of Vegan Protein Powder or whey isolate
- 1 scoop of a Greens Powder (Genuine Health) or any greens powder

Directions

With a hand mixer or blender mix all ingredients together. Enjoy!

Helpful tip:

People who begin their day with a protein breakfast are less likely to overeat at the end of the day and are more likely to maintain a healthy weight. Protein helps to ramp up your metabolism. When you eat protein, something called the thermic effect of food (TEF) takes place. Your body uses more calories to digest, absorb, transport and metabolize your food helping you burn more calories. Whoo-hoo!

DID YOU KNOW?

Research shows that women with essential fatty acid deficiencies often experience PMS. Prostaglandins are vital hormone like compounds that act as transient hormones which balance your body's EFA flow. To increase your essential fatty acids try adding a tablespoon of flax, borage, or evening of primrose oils to your smoothies (especially in the last half of your cycle).

nutritional nibble...

It is difficult to get the vitamins and minerals you need when you are under any amount of stress. And yes, PMS can be stressful for many of us! When stressed, our cells switch into high gear and use up the nutrition we take in at an accelerated rate, just to function. It is important that we keep up by providing our bodies with higher levels of nutrition all day long, focusing on vitamins C, B and E. This is easy to do. Just begin by boosting up the nutritional status of your breakfast by adding in some highly nutritious greens. Smoothies are great because you can easily add spinach, kale or broccoli and you won't even know it's there…really. Another easy way to get more greens is to add a green powder supplement to your daily diet. There are many brands out there but some that we like and that are available at most larger grocery stores are Genuine Health, Greens Plus and Barleans.

Mighty Maca Smoothie: Serves 1

This smoothie makes a great mid afternoon snack and is much healthier for PMS then a caffeine laden beverage, but will still provide that afternoon pick me up with the added hormone balancing benefits of Maca.

Ingredients

- 1 ½ cups almond milk (unsweetened)
- 1 cup orange juice
    (or slice of organic orange, including rind if using a Vitamix)
- 1 tsp Maca powder
- ¼ avocado
- 3 cups of baby spinach
- 4 dates (to sweeten)

Directions

Blend all ingredients together in a blender and enjoy.

nutritional nibbles...

Maca may just be the perfect food for PMS or on those days when you need an extra boost of energy. Maca Root Powder nourishes the adrenal glands and balances hormones. And if Peruvian warriors used Maca root before battle to increase their strength and endurance shouldn't you do the same when fighting PMS?

One cup of spinach contains 20% of your RDA of fibre, phytonutrients, antioxidants Vitamin C and E, and 337% of your RDA of Vitamin A, is high in calcium and magnesium and can help you fight infection. No wonder Popeye was a fan!

DID YOU KNOW?

Organic spinach is highly recommended. Lettuce is one food that is best to eat organic because of its high pesticide content. Give your liver a break from having to detox pesticides and go organic for your leafy greens so that you can reap the nutritional rewards that they provide.

Many women who experience PMS symptoms are deficient in calcium and magnesium. Increasing calcium and magnesium sources in your diet (see the fantastic recipes in this book!) can reduce bloating, cramping, food cravings and improve your mood. Hair element analysis can be useful to determine if you have a calcium or magnesium deficiency. This non-invasive test involves sending a small sample of hair to a lab where it is analyzed for its mineral content. The results can be used to create a supplement plan tailored to suit your needs.

Dr. Jane Goehner, ND Dr.

Consult your nutritionist or naturopathic doctor to see if a calcium magnesium supplement is appropriate for you.

Say hello to our little friend…fibre! Rich in fibre and extremely low in fat, this soup makes an excellent anti PMS meal. High fibre foods enhance estrogen excretion and are thought to help improve hormonal balance and decrease mood imbalances.
In addition, a diet low in fat (especially in saturated fat) also reduces estrogen levels as well as many PMS symptoms, such as emotional changes (crying at that Hallmark ad again?) and bloating.

Ingredients

- 1 tbsp coconut oil or grapeseed oil
- 1 large yellow onion, sliced
- 2 carrots, diced
- 2 cloves garlic
- 1 tsp ground ginger
- 2 tsp ground cumin
- 2 tsp ground coriander seeds
- 1 cup red lentils (dry), rinsed
- 28 oz (420 g) canned tomatoes
- 2 sweet potatoes, chopped
- 6 cups vegetable stock (read ingredient list)
- freshly ground pepper and sea salt to taste
- 2 – 4 tbsp Chia Seeds
- Greek style yogurt to serve (optional)

NUTRITIONAL NIBBLE

Chia seeds are a great way to add fibre to your diet. Add them to soups and smoothies, or sprinkle them on yogurt for a tasty way to increase your fibre intake. And don't forget to have plenty of vegetables which is another healthy way to increase fibre, remove toxins, increase nutrients and decrease cravings.

Directions

Peel and crush garlic. Set aside. (Leaving crushed or minced garlic for at least 5 – 10 minutes after crushing helps maximize its health-protective effects.) Heat oil in a large non-stick saucepan over medium heat. Add onion and cook for 3 minutes, stirring occasionally. Add stock, lentils, canned tomatoes, carrots, potato, ginger, cumin, coriander, salt and pepper, and bring to boil. Cover pot and let simmer for 25 minutes over medium heat. Add garlic and let simmer for another 5 minutes.

Purée soup in a blender or use a hand immersion blender to process soup until smooth. Add Chia Seeds and mix well. Spoon soup into bowls and top with a generous dollop of yogurt.

Wait …doesn't salt cause water retention?

Not this kind! Sea salt is loaded with minerals! And mineral loaded salts actually help to balance our electrolytes and release retained water. Sea salt may also prevent cramping. Sea salt should be damp and grey looking. This tells you it hasn't been processed and/or bleached and still retains its mineral content. Minerals are tough enough to get into our diets, so we need all we can get! You can find Celtic Sea Salt at most health food stores.

Want to be less of a "B"?

If you want to control your mood and more importantly, your mood swings, you need to make sure your diet includes B vitamins, especially Vitamin B6.

What is the big deal with Vitamin B6?

It plays an important role in the synthesis of the neurotransmitter dopamine. This contributes to our physical and emotional well-being by helping to improve our mood and outlook which is very important at a time of the month when everything and everyone are potentially annoying you!

Vitamin B6 is also connected to hormone balance and water shifts in women and helps to maintain the potassium, phosphorus and sodium balance in our bodies. It acts as a natural diuretic to help control bloating.

Vitamin B6 may also help relieve other PMS symptoms, including breast tenderness, depression, and anxiety. It promotes the absorption of zinc and magnesium which are an integral part of an anti-PMS diet. Supplementation may help – especially at those times of the month when you are more stressed!

Be all that you can "B"!

Not many foods have super high amounts of B6 because it is often lost in cooking, refining or processing of foods… another reason to avoid processed foods!

The best food sources of vitamin B6 are: meat (especially organ meats such as liver) and whole grains, such as wheat and wheat germ. Fish, poultry, egg yolk, soybeans and other dried beans, peanuts, and walnuts also provide this important vitamin. Veggie and fruit sources include: bananas, prunes, potatoes, cauliflower, cabbage, collard, turnip, mustard greens, garlic, mushrooms, spinach, bell peppers, avocados, chickpeas, lentils, and bananas.

Are your Adrenals letting you down?

There are many interesting books that will open your eyes to just how important the tiny little adrenal glands are to your hormonal health. If your PMS symptoms are getting worse as the years go by, you might want to consider looking at your adrenal health. Talk to your Naturopath and/or Nutritionist for more guidance.

Be all that you can "B" Avocado Salad: Serves 2

Ingredients

- 1 large avocado, peeled, pitted and diced
- 1 cup cucumber
- ¼ cup Spanish onion
- handful of grape tomatoes
- dash of balsamic vinegar
- 1 tbsp cold pressed olive oil
- sunflower seeds, to taste
- salt and freshly ground pepper, to taste
- optional – 1 tbsp crumbled feta cheese

Directions

Mix avocado, onion, and tomatoes into bowl. Drizzle balsamic vinegar and olive oil on top and sprinkle with sunflower seeds to add crunch. Finish with some sea salt and pepper to taste.

ABOUT THIS RECIPE

This salad is loaded with fibre rich avocadoes, high in vitamin B6 which you now know is a crucial mood regulator and very helpful in the fight against PMS. Eat your way to a better mood, and say good-bye to the "B" in you and hello to deliciousness. Dive in, those around you will be happy you did!

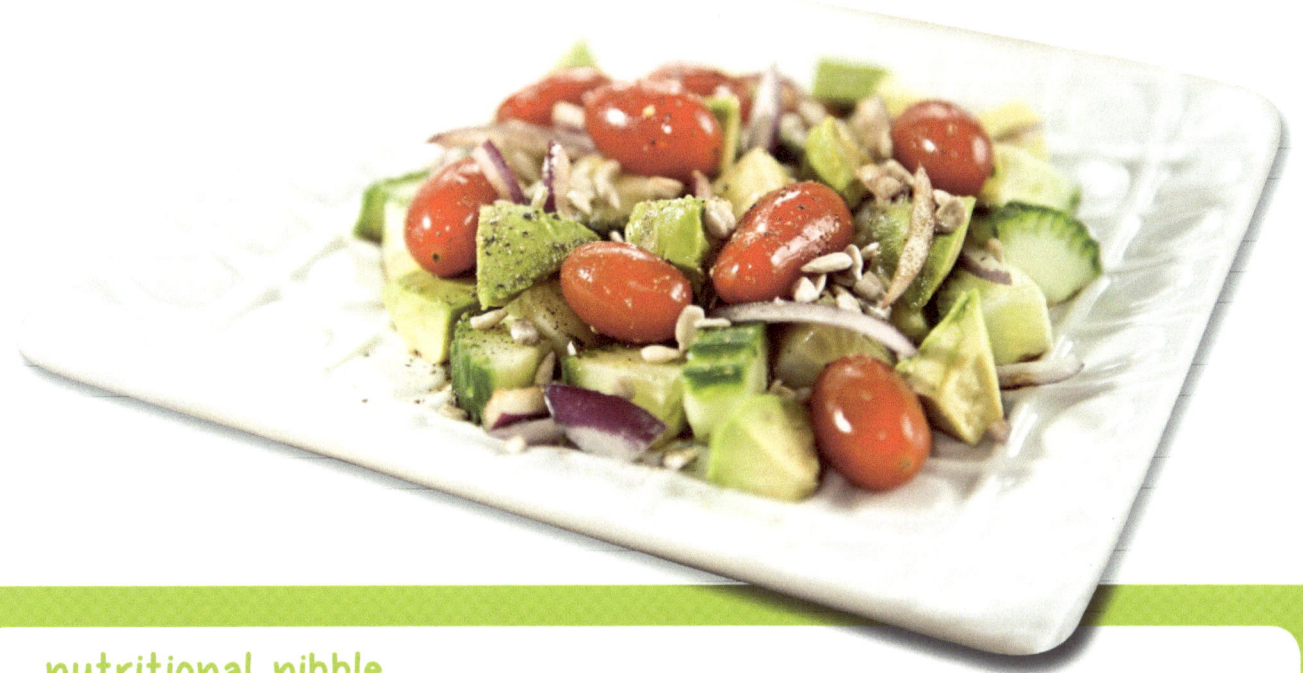

nutritional nibble...

Avocadoes are loaded with dietary fibre, EFAs and vitamin B6 which play an important role in an anti PMS diet. This vitamin does more than regulate mood. It also metabolizes amino acids (protein), fat and carbohydrates and helps to build red blood cells – especially important during that time of the month when women can become anemic. In addition, the high fibre content in avocados will keep you feeling full and its essential fatty acids will help keep your skin glowing and your hormones in balance.

Isn't it ironic?

The time we need iron the most is the time of the month when we deplete it the most. Iron contributes to mood, energy, thyroid health, and our overall well-being so balancing this mineral is key; it is not good to have too much or too little. According to dieticians of Canada we should aim for about 18 mg of iron daily.

Where can you get it?

- Animal sources (called heme iron) are more easily absorbed by the body – meat, fish and poultry
- Plant sources (called non-heme iron) – dried beans, lentils, and peas, and some vegetables

Iron friends:

Best plant sources:	Best meat choices:
spirulina (1tsp = 5 mg)	liver (3 oz = 5.8 mg) (use only organic from a trusted farm)
spinach (1/2 cup = 2 mg)	corned beef – 3.5 oz = 4.3 mg
tomato puree (4 oz = 3.9 mg)	veal, ham, beef, pork – 3.5 oz = 3.5 mg
lima beans (1/2 cup = 2.2)	sardines – 3.5 oz = 2.9 mg
morel mushrooms	venison
almonds – 1/2 cup 3.4 mg	Turkey (dark meat) – 3.5 oz = 2.3 mg
tofu	oysters
lentils (4 oz = 3 mg)	seafood (shrimp, crab, scallops)
baked beans – 1/2 cup = 2.3 mg	
tempeh, beans (1/2 cup = 3.9 mg)	
blackstrap molasses (1 tbsp = 4 mg)	
amaranth, teff	
quinoa (4 oz = 4 mg)	
sesame seeds	
pumpkin seeds (1 oz = 4.2 mg)	
oatmeal and other fortified cereals	
prune juice – 1 cup = 5.3 mg	

Iron foes:

Polyphenols in coffee and tea will bind to iron, making it more difficult to absorb. Calcium also hinders absorption…so consider eating higher calcium foods about 30 minutes away from your high iron foods. Soak your beans and grains first to break down the phytic acid that inhibits iron absorption. When it comes to bread, choose sourdough varieties; the fermentation process breaks down the iron inhibitors.

Kale is the new super food that many health gurus are buzzing about. While many of them are are excited by its super nutrients, many more of us aren't as thrilled by its unique taste. Try this salad and we guarantee you will be a kale convert. It is wonderfully tasty and makes a nice complement to a warm soup for a fall or winter meal.

Ingredients

- 2 large bunches of curly kale, chopped well
- 1 yellow, orange or red pepper, chopped
- ½ cup olive oil
- ⅓ cup apple cider vinegar
- ¼ cup peanuts or almonds
- 2 tbsp honey
- 1 tsp sea salt
- Cayenne pepper to taste
- ¼ peanuts to top or almonds

Directions

Mix chopped kale with peppers. Blend olive oil, vinegar, honey, sea salt, cayenne pepper and ⅓ cup peanuts or almonds. Mix into salad just before serving. Sprinkle with peanuts or almonds and sea salt to taste.

nutritional nibble...

Hail Kale! Kale is extremely high in antioxidants scoring a 1770, the highest of the vegetables, on the ORAC (oxygen radical absorbance capacity) scale, a scale that measures oxidant power. Chock full of minerals such as calcium and iron, and vitamins A, C, K, this super vegetable has about 10 times the beta carotene of broccoli. Kale also releases sulphoraphane when the vegetable is chewed or chopped, triggering the liver to remove free radicals and other chemicals that may cause DNA damage. This boosts the body's detoxifying enzymes and may also fight cancer. PMS has been linked to faulty liver fat metabolism. Lipotropics found in kale decongest the liver making the job of processing hormones easier and helps to battle PMS!

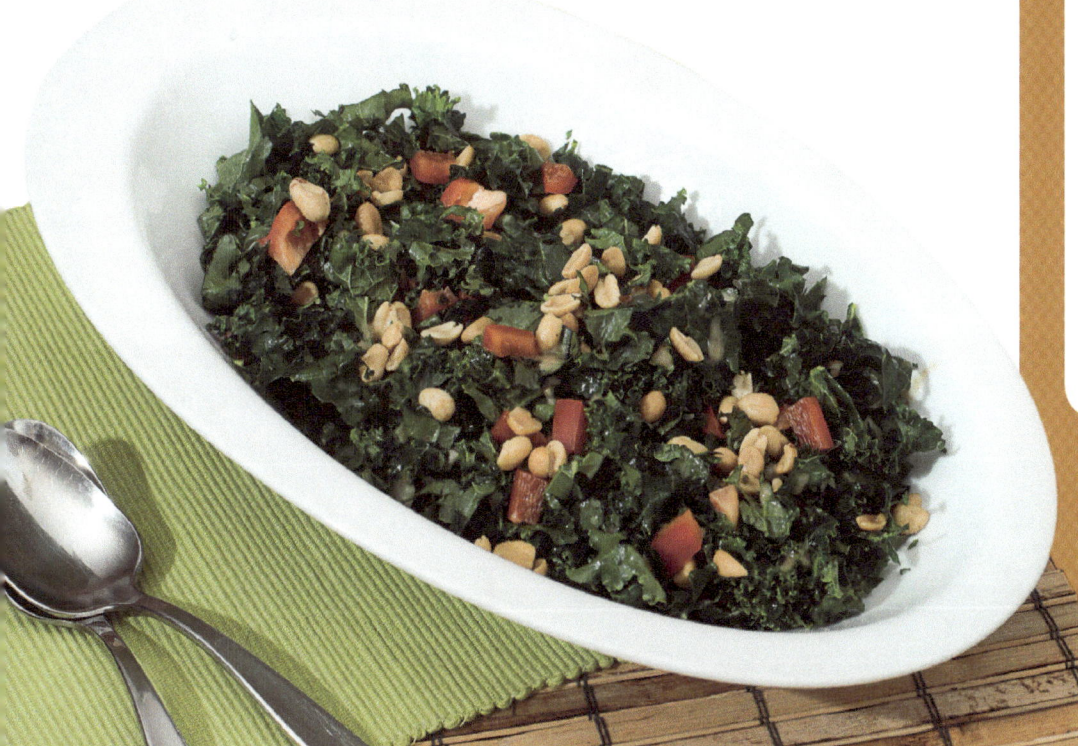

Ingredients

- 6 cups baby spinach
- 2 tbsp red onion, diced
- ¼ red pepper, chopped
- 2 hard-boiled, hormone-free eggs, peeled and chopped
- 1 tbsp feta cheese, crumbled
- 1 tbsp dried sulphite free cranberries or chopped apple

Directions

Dressing: blend 1 – 2 tablespoons of apple cider vinegar, ¼ cup extra virgin olive oil, ½ teaspoons of mustard powder, maple syrup, salt and pepper to taste.

Mix all ingredients together in a large bowl.
Top with 1 – 2 tablespoons of the dressing.

○ RECIPE TIP ○

To avoid that greyish tint that sometimes surrounds the yolk on a hard-boiled egg try this: place eggs in a saucepan and cover with water. Bring to a boil and then turn the heat off and put a lid on the saucepan. Leave for at least 5 minutes to finish cooking through. Voilà …beautiful yellows!

about this recipe…

We all know Popeye loved his greens and if Popeye were a woman he would have been a happy camper. And while Popeye knew that dark leafy greens are packed with iron and nutrients he may not have realized that by combining the spinach with the 'rich' Vitamin C foods, your body will be able to use the iron more effectively. This salad does that for you! Add any of the following ingredients to any dark green leafy salad for better iron absorption: strawberries, kiwi, peppers, broccoli, cauliflower, tomatoes, or fresh squeezed lemon or lime. So get pumped!

nutritional nibble…

Apple cider vinegar has many health benefits but the one we like most is that apple cider vinegar significantly improved insulin sensitivity in insulin-resistant subjects. Begin your meals with a salad topped with apple cider vinegar for help with managing blood sugar.

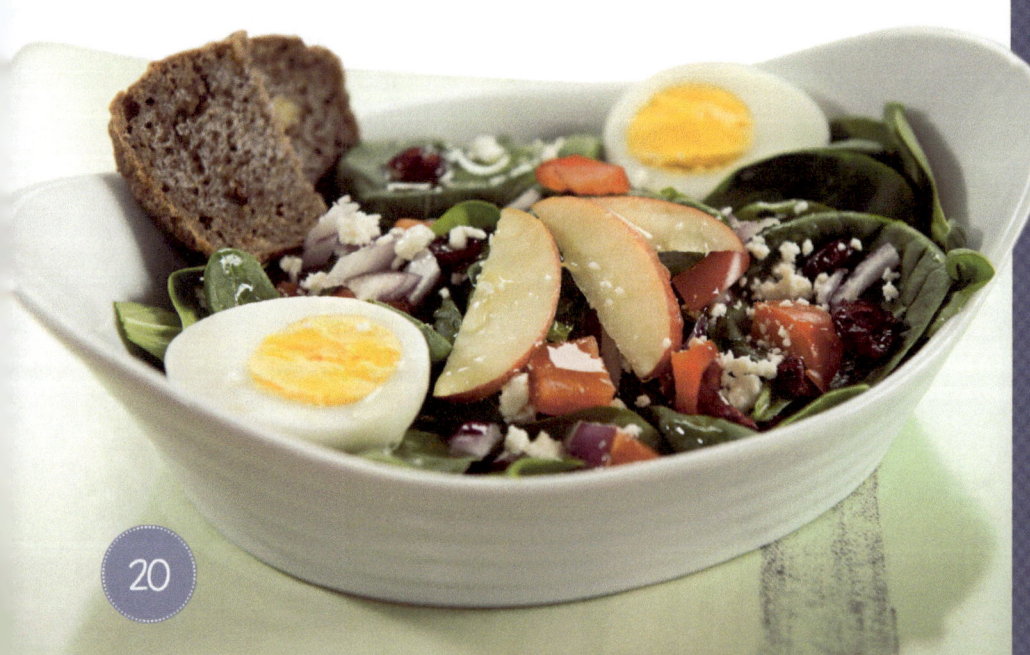

Many of the store bought veggie burgers are loaded with soy and additives that are not so PMS friendly. This vegetarian recipe is full of beans which are of course are loaded with fibre, perfect for the PMS eating plan. It isn't always easy to get the 35 grams of daily fibre that our bodies need but this recipe will help you do that.

Ingredients

- 2 cups cooked beans
- 1 cup squash, mashed
- 1 carrot, chopped
- ½ onion, chopped
- 1 clove garlic, finely diced
- ½ cup miso liquid or stock to moisten patties (optional)
- 1 egg or 1 tbsp ground flax seeds mixed into 3 tbsp water to bind
- 1 tbsp fresh herbs like coriander, parsley, fennel, cumin, mint and/or garlic
- ½ cup quinoa
- sunflower seeds

HELPFUL TIP

Herbs are much more than a pretty garnish. Parsley is high in magnesium!

Directions

Mash up the beans. Mix in other ingredients and form into patties. Bake for 30 minutes at 400°F until brown or you can melt 1 tablespoon of coconut oil in a pan and fry until lightly browned. Flip over and cook second side. Serve topped with guacamole or salsa.

nutritional nibble...

Adding more vegetarian meals into your weekly menu will help you to help you lower your saturated fat intake, an important component to the anti PMS diet. Vegetarian meals are easy on the budget and great for your overall health. Just make sure you enjoy SMART vegetarian meals that provide complete proteins and are glycemic index friendly meals. For a complete protein, use the following combinations: rice + beans, rice + seeds/nuts, corn + beans, beans + nuts/seeds.

Vegetarian Dhal: Serves 6 - 8

Dhal is an Indian term for a thick, soup like stew made from different legumes. This is nourishing and easy to digest and is a staple in Ayurvedic cooking.

Ingredients

- 2 tbsp coconut oil or ghee
- 1 medium onion, chopped
- 3 tbsp fresh ginger, peeled, grated
- 3 cloves garlic, chopped
- 3 cups water or vegetable stock
- 1 cup dried red lentils, rinsed and drained
- 1-2 tsp each of turmeric and cumin
- ½ tsp cayenne
- ¾ cup fresh cilantro, washed, stemmed, chopped
- 3 plum tomatoes
- Sea salt to taste

Directions

In saucepan over medium heat, saute onions, garlic, and ginger in coconut oil until onions are soft. Add turmeric and cumin and saute lightly. Pour in the water or broth and then add lentils. Increase heat to high and cook until the mixture comes to a boil. Reduce heat and simmer, stirring occasionally, until the lentils are tender, about 15 minutes. Mix or whisk the mixture well until it is thick and creamy looking. Add the tomatoes and salt to taste and simmer for an additional 10 minutes. Top with cilantro and gently stir in just before serving.

You can serve this alone as a starter or serve with brown basmati rice or quinoa.

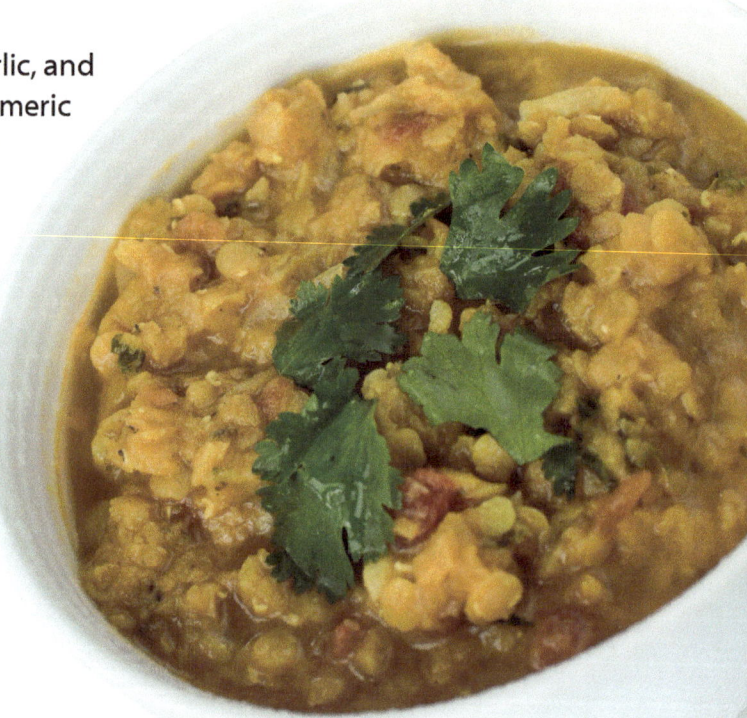

Did you know?

Turmeric helps combat inflammation. Inflammation is responsible for a host of diseases (heart disease, cancer, etc.) and contributes to joint pain and body aches, and yes, weight gain! Adding more turmeric to your diet may help relieve your aches and pains at that time of month when you're experiencing discomfort. Some studies show that it even helps reduce plaque build-up in the brain, a major contributor to Alzheimer's. So spice it up and reap major health benefits!

Looks like turkey isn't just for Thanksgiving anymore! Try this delicious twist on lasagna, PMS style. Gobble, gobble.

Ingredients

- 1 tsp water or grapeseed oil
- 500 g ground hormone free turkey or chicken
- 1 small onion, finely diced
- 1 garlic clove, minced
- 227 g pkg sliced button mushrooms, chopped
- ½ tsp dried oregano
- ½ tsp dried basil
- 398 mL can tomato sauce
- 2 tsp sucanat sugar
- 3 10 inch brown rice flour tortillas
- 4 cups baby spinach
- 2 cups shredded mozzarella-cheddar cheese mix or Daiya (dairy free) cheese

Directions

Preheat oven to 350°F. Lightly spray a 9 inch pie plate with oil. Heat a non-stick frying pan over medium. Add oil or water, then turkey. Sauté meat until no pink remains, about 3 minutes. Add onion, garlic, mushrooms and herbs. Cook until onion is soft, about 3 minutes. Stir in tomato sauce and sugar. Gently boil until sauce reduces slightly, 5 minutes. Assemble lasagna by placing a tortilla on the bottom of prepared pie plate. Spread 1 ⅓ cups sauce in an even layer over tortilla. Scatter 1 ⅓ cups spinach, then ⅔ cup of cheese mix overtop, pressing down gently on the tortilla as you layer. Repeat with remaining tortillas, sauce, spinach and cheese. (The spinach will cook down as it bakes.) Bake in centre of oven, uncovered, until cheese is melted, about 20 minutes. Let stand for 5 minutes before cutting into wedges.

nutritional nibble...

Sucanat sugar is simple and unrefined sugar. The beautiful white sugar we are used to seeing has been processed to be more appealing by the use of sulphur dioxide. In order to make it "pretty" virtually all the minerals are refined right out of the sugar. If you use more natural sources of foods, including sugar, you will get the right balance of minerals so your body doesn't need to draw the 'missing' minerals from your body to be able to digest that food. Eat your foods whole because whole foods contain the right balance of nutrients and minerals for you! Sucanat may not be as pretty to look at (it is brown and grainy looking) but at least it has some vitamins and minerals left! It tastes slightly like molasses.

23

Lemon Chicken and Feta: Serves 4

We love Greek food, but typical restaurant type Greek dishes are laden with heavy oils and cheeses. This dish gives you all the Mediterranean flavour you love with the health benefits of a more traditional Mediterranean diet. It is simple and delicious and your whole family will love it. Opa!

Ingredients

- 1 lemon
- 1 tbsp (15 mL) chopped fresh dill or ½ tsp (2 mL) dried dillweed
- 4 oz (125 g) block of feta, preferably light
- 4 skinless, organic, hormone free boneless chicken breasts or tempeh
- grapeseed oil
- 1 bunch broccoli
- ¼ cup (50 mL) whole skin-on almonds (optional)

Directions

Preheat oven to 400°F (200°C). Line a large baking sheet with parchment paper or lightly oil. Finely grate peel from lemon into a bowl. Stir in dill and pinches of salt. Cut feta into thick wedges. Cut chicken breasts in half horizontally. Place feta and chicken on parchment. Lightly drizzle both with olive oil, then sprinkle with half the seasoning mix. Roast in centre of preheated oven for 10 minutes. Meanwhile, cut broccoli into large florets. When chicken has roasted for 10 minutes, add broccoli and almonds. Sprinkle with remaining seasoning and stir. Continue roasting until chicken is cooked through, from 10 to 15 more minutes. Squeeze juice from lemon over top.

Did you know?

According to research done at the University of California, almonds are more easily digested after roasting. The coating on the almond is rigid making it harder for the stomach to breakdown during the digestion process so that a large portion of raw almond tissue is never fully digested. Roasting almonds changes their texture, making them easier to digest and, since almond tissue is lost through the digestion process, roasted almonds may release more nutrients in the body than raw ones. Less almond tissue is lost through the digestion process so roasted almonds may release more nutrients in the body than raw ones. Just be careful…most commercially roasted almonds are loaded with unhealthy and rancid oils. If you roast them yourself, like in this recipe, you can enjoy the health benefits of almonds, along with their delicious flavour.

NUTRITIONAL NIBBLE

This recipe is considered an anti PMS recipe because it is high in calcium and Vitamin E and low glycemic.

Where's the beef? Unlike the lady from the popular commercial of years ago we guarantee that with this tasty meatloaf, made with ground turkey instead of beef, you won't be asking that question.

Ingredients

- 2 tbsp grapeseed oil
- 1 red bell pepper, finely diced
- 1 yellow bell pepper, finely diced
- 5 cloves garlic, smashed to a paste with coarse salt
- ½ tsp red pepper flakes
- Kosher salt and freshly ground pepper
- 1 large egg, lightly beaten
- 1 tbsp finely chopped fresh thyme
- ¼ cup chopped fresh parsley
- 1 ½ pounds ground hormone and antibiotic free turkey (90 percent lean)
- 1 cup wheat free bread crumbs
- ½ cup grated Daiya cheese
- ¾ cup ketchup and/or salsa
- ¼ cup balsamic vinegar

DID YOU KNOW?

The majority of animals raised for consumption are given estrogen in order to make them grow bigger and faster. This estrogen is then passed along when you eat the meat. According to Samuel Epstein, Founder of the Cancer Prevention Coalition, meat treated with hormones increases breast cancer risk. High estrogen levels are also one of the causes of PMS. In order to lower estrogen exposure from meats, eat meat that was raised without the use of hormones.

Directions

Preheat the oven to 425°F. Heat the oil in a large pan over high heat. Add the bell peppers, garlic paste and ¼ teaspoon red pepper flakes. Season with salt and pepper and cook until the vegetables are almost soft, about 5 minutes. Set aside to cool.

Whisk the egg and fresh herbs in a large bowl. Add the turkey, bread crumbs, grated cheese, ½ cup ketchup/salsa and the cooled vegetables; mix until just combined.

Gently press the mixture into a 9-by-5-inch loaf pan. Whisk the remaining ¼ cup ketchup, ¼ cup balsamic vinegar and ¼ teaspoon red pepper flakes in a small bowl; brush the mixture over the entire loaf. Bake for 1 hour. Let rest for 10 minutes before slicing.

Serve with a large green salad for a complete meal.

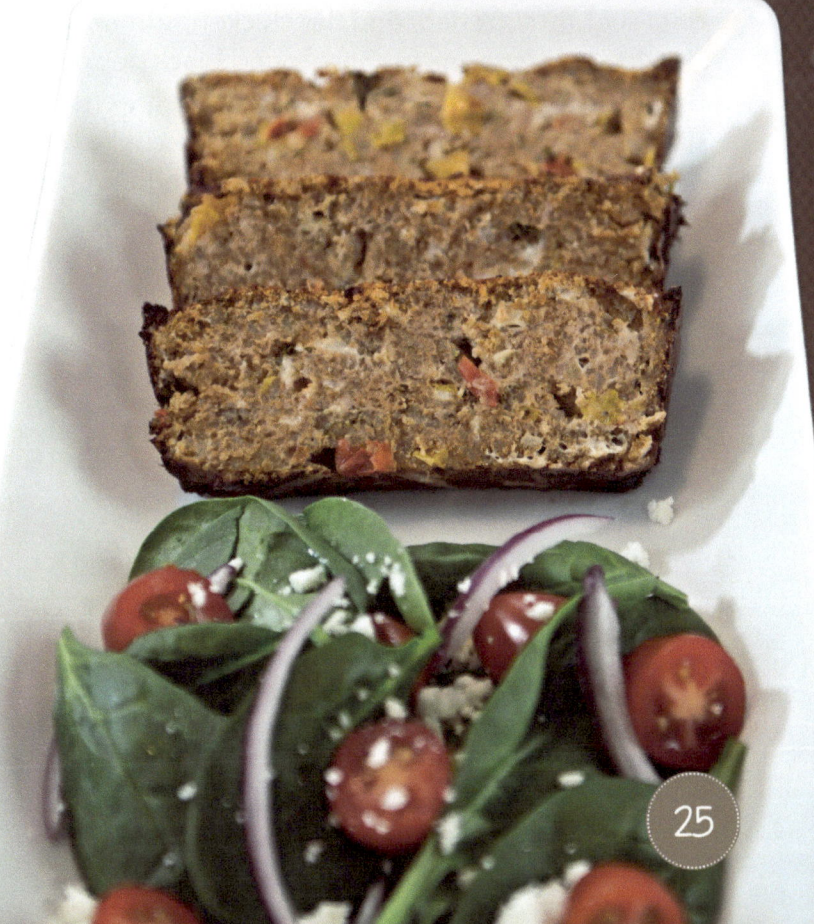

Nothing is more satisfying on a cold day then a warm bowl of chilli. This is another high fibre meal. (Do you see a theme here?) High in protein and flavour you'll want to make this your tailgating, football party standard, even when you don't have PMS.

Ingredients

- 2 tbsp coconut oil
- 1 tbsp minced garlic
- ¾ cup diced onion
- 1 pound skinless, boneless chicken breasts, finely chopped
- 1 tbsp ground cumin
- 1 tbsp dried oregano
- ½ tsp ground white pepper
- pinch of red pepper flakes
- sea salt and freshly ground pepper
- 1 pound collard greens, stemmed and roughly chopped (about 5 cups)
- 1 ½ cups chopped green chillies, optional
- 1 quart low-sodium chicken broth
- 2 15-ounce can navy beans, drained and rinsed
- ½ bunch fresh cilantro, chopped
- light sour cream, chopped tomatoes and/or lime wedges, for garnish (optional)

DID YOU KNOW?

Extra Virgin Olive oil is best for salad. When heated, the oil breaks down and is no longer beneficial to the body. Try grapeseed or coconut oil instead for cooking.

Directions

In a saucepan, heat the oil over medium heat. Add the garlic and onion. Cook for 2 to 3 minutes, until slightly softened. Add the chicken, cumin, oregano, pepper and flakes. Season with salt and 1 to 2 teaspoons freshly ground black pepper. Cook, stirring, until the chicken is slightly browned, 3 to 4 minutes. Add the collard greens and cook, stirring occasionally, until they are slightly wilted, about 5 minutes. Add the chillies and chicken broth and bring to a boil, stirring occasionally. Reduce the heat to medium-low. Cook, stirring occasionally, for approximately 20 minutes, until slightly thickened. Stir in the beans and cook for another 10 minutes. Stir in the cilantro. Transfer the chilli to bowls and garnish with light sour cream, chopped tomatoes and/or lime wedges, if desired.

nutritional nibble...

You grow up believing that chicken stock is good for you and before we began to rely on commercially prepared broth laden with unhealthy ingredients such as trans fats, MSG, yeasts and gluten, that was true. If you suffer from celiac disease, gluten intolerances, candida, yeast overgrowth or are dealing with other health issues, you may want to omit commercial broths from your diet, or make your own. However, if you don't want to make your own, just be sure to look for yeast and gluten free varieties available at health food stores and some of the larger chains in the health food sections. Check your labels before you buy!

We all know that fish is good for us. Yet many of us like our fish with batter, beer, and chips…which is not so healthy. We also know that preparing it 'sans' batter and getting the whole family to enjoy it can be a challenge. So we've met that challenge and come up with this flavourful compromise by using a little breading and some healthy almonds to boost the flavour and nutrition while keeping it family and PMS friendly. The best part is there's no deep fryer required!

Ingredients

- 2 pounds halibut fillets, cut in 8 pieces
- 2 hormone-free eggs
- ¼ cup water
- ¼ cup brown rice flour
- ½ tsp salt
- ¼ tsp pepper
- 1 cup almonds, processed to flour in coffee grinder
- 1 cup dry bread crumbs, preferably gluten free
- 1 tbsp sesame seeds
- ½ cup coconut oil
- salsa

Directions

Rinse the fish and pat dry with paper towel. Mix the eggs with a small amount of water. Mix the flour with salt and pepper and transfer to plate. Mix almonds, sesame seeds and bread crumbs and place on plate. Coat fish in flour, then egg, then crumb mixture. Melt coconut oil and then brown each side of the fish in a pan. Or, bake in oven at 400°F for 10 – 15 minutes or until cooked. Serve with guacamole or salsa.

nutritional nibble…

Most of us now know that fish is high in omega 3s, the powerful fatty acids with a myriad of health benefits, but did you know that some types of fish contain higher levels of these beneficial fatty acids than others? Fish and shellfish with higher omega 3 content that are also low in mercury include: anchovy, capelin, char, herring, Atlantic mackerel, mullet, pollock (Boston bluefish), salmon, smelt, rainbow trout, lake whitefish, blue crab, shrimp, clams, mussels and oysters.

According to the Division of Environmental Health, Halibut is safe to eat once a week. If you have concerns about the mercury content of your fish, information on types of fish and how often they can be safely eaten is available at the following link: *http://www.doh.wa.gov/ehp/oehas/fish/fishchart.html*.

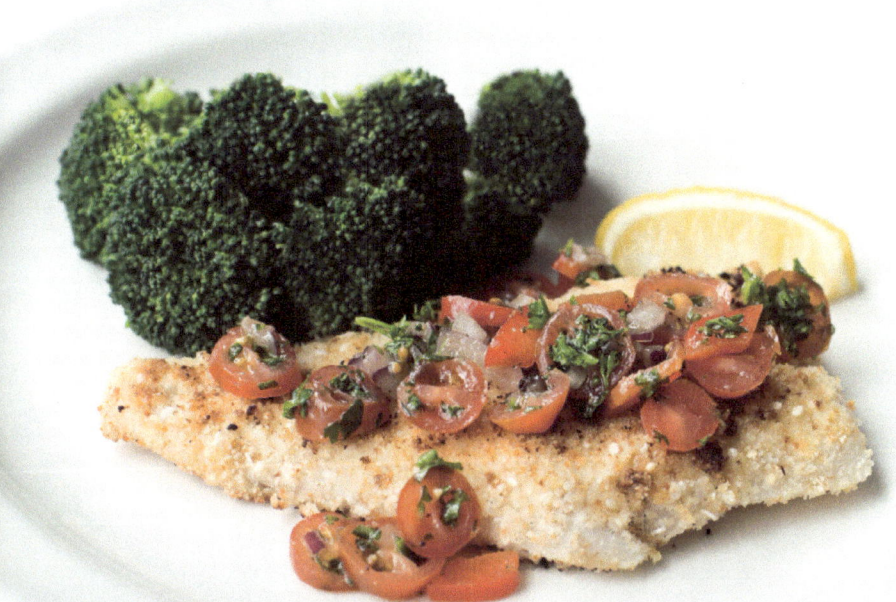

This recipe is a wonderful meal for a week night in the summer. It is so simple and easy. You can prepare the entire meal the night before, leave it in the fridge, and then simply cook the shrimp and toss with the dressing and cabbage mix when ready to eat.

Ingredients

- 2 tbsp lime juice
- 2 tsp Bragg's Liquid Aminos Soy Sauce
- 2 tsp toasted sesame oil
- ½ tsp agave nectar
- 3 cups thinly sliced cabbage (napa)
- 1 small red or orange pepper, thinly sliced
- 2 tbsp rice flour
- ¼ tsp sea salt
- ½ tsp freshly ground pepper
- ½ tsp five-spice powder
- 3 tbsp sulfite-free shredded coconut
- 10 oz raw shrimp peeled and deveined
- 1 tbsp coconut oil
- 1 jalapeno pepper, seeded and mince

Directions

Whisk lime juice, Bragg's soy sauce, sesame oil and agave in a large bowl until mixed. Add cabbage and bell pepper and toss to combine. Combine rice flour, salt, pepper, coconut and five-spice powder in medium bowl. Add shrimp and toss to coat. Heat coconut oil in a large non-stick skillet over medium high heat. Add the shrimp and cook, stirring often, until they are pink and curled, 3 – 4 minutes. Add jalapeno and cook until the shrimp are cooked through, about 1 minute more. Serve the slaw topped with the shrimp.

NUTRITIONAL NIBBLE

Shrimp is high in zinc, an important mineral that many are deficient in. Mineral deficiencies contribute to a host of health problems including PMS. Shrimp are also high in iron and selenium which give hair its healthy glow and mood boosting vitamin B6.

Did you know?

Regular soy sauce contains wheat gluten. As mentioned, many people are intolerant to gluten. If that's you, try Braggs Liquid Aminos, a gluten free soy sauce with no preservatives, wheat or artificial colours. This healthier version of soy sauce can be found in many grocery stores (health food section) and health food stores.

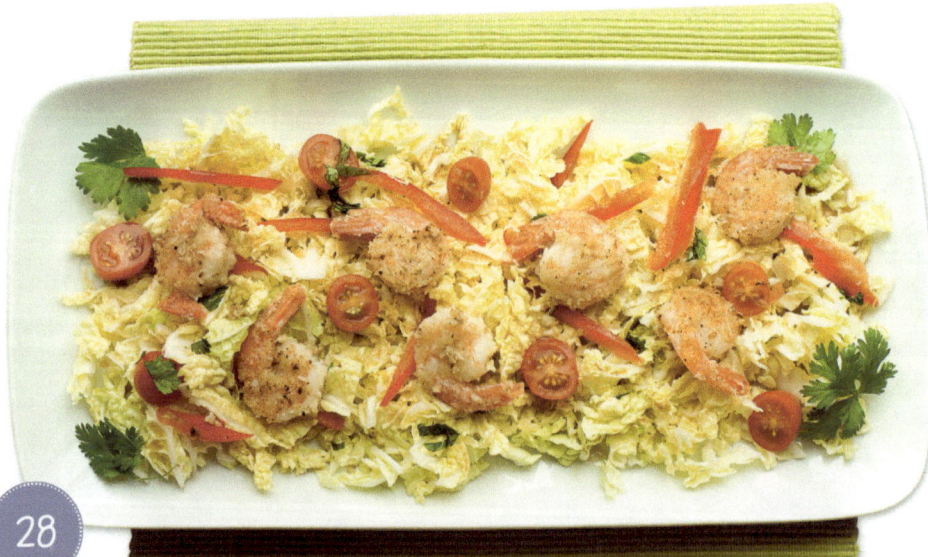

Sometimes you just need hearty pasta to fill you up and provide you with good energy. This recipe is a healthier alternative to traditional gluten filled pasta because it uses quinoa, a whole grain that is higher in protein, and gluten free. The tuna, also high in protein, lowers the glycemic index of the meal. So mangia, mangia!

Ingredients

- ¼ cup grapeseed oil or coconut oil
- 2 cloves garlic, crushed
- ¼ to ½ tsp hot red pepper flakes, to taste
- 1 tsp anchovy paste
- 1 can Italian plum tomatoes
- 1 cup chopped leafy green like spinach or kale
- 1 tsp agave nectar or sweetener of choice
- coarse sea salt and pepper to taste
- 12 oz water-packed tuna, drained
- 4 tbsp chopped fresh parsley
- quinoa pasta

NUTRITIONAL NIBBLE

While tuna fish is fine in moderation, it is not something you should consume more than once a month due to its high mercury content. For the lowest mercury levels choose light tuna instead of the white albacore variety.

Directions

Heat the oil in a skillet and add the garlic. Fry on medium-low heat until golden and then add the hot red pepper flakes and stir instantly to keep from burning. Add the anchovy paste and stir to dissolve with a wooden spoon. Add the tomatoes, agave and salt and pepper. Mix and simmer on medium heat for 15 to 20 minutes.

Add the tuna, breaking it up with the spoon. Add some of the parsley and cook for 10 minutes more. Cook pasta as per the package directions. Pour the sauce over the pasta, mix well, and sprinkle with the remaining parsley. Serve immediately.

Note: Gluten free pasta is best the day you cook it so make just enough for the meal.

Did you know?

To lower the GI of grains like pasta which have a higher gylcemic rating than whole grains, (sorry Chef Boyardee) you can add balsamic vinegar (or lemon juice) to them. Balsamic vinegar not only adds flavour it also slows down the rate at which the carbs and glucose hit your blood-stream, lowering the overall glycemic load of the meal. Also, be sure to cook your pasta al dente because it will take longer for your body to break down the starch, placing it lower on the glycemic scale than pasta that is overcooked. So pass the vinegar please!

Raw Chocolate Pudding: Serves 2 - 4

If you've had chocolate four times already and it's only noon… it must be PMS. Chocolate cravings are part and parcel of PMS but they don't have to be unhealthy chocolate choices. This pudding gets its creamy texture from avocados! You won't be able to taste them but your body will certainly appreciate the healthy fat and fibre they contain. It is so good, be sure to make enough to share!

Ingredients

- 2 soft bananas
- 1 soft avocado
- 1 tbsp agave nectar or raw honey (or stevia for a sugar free version)
- 2 tbsp raw cacao powder (carob powder if you are avoiding chocolate)
- optional – 1 tbsp almond butter for a protein boost and nuttier flavour!
- optional toppings – coconut or nuts

Directions

Blend banana, avocado, cacao powder and sweetener of choice until smooth. (A Vita Mix works best but food processors are good too.) Scoop pudding into small bowls and then refrigerate for at least 1 hour. Top with coconut or chopped walnuts.

Enjoy!

nutritional nibble...

Cacao is a good source of the minerals magnesium, sulphur, calcium, iron, zinc, copper, potassium, and manganese; plus some of the B Vitamins. It not only helps satisfy chocolate cravings, the pure stuff actually helps fight PMS! Yay, finally we're justified in eating it! For those who get migraines or other negative symptoms from eating chocolate, try raw cacao. The raw version is in its natural, unprocessed, and unaltered state which is rich in nutrients and healthy. Give it a try! Raw cacao can be found in health food stores in the form of powder or nibs.

Did you know?

Did you know that we actually crave chocolate for a reason? Usually chocolate cravings are a sign that we are low in the mineral magnesium. So how do we increase our magnesium levels… yes…chocolate!!! Before you jump off the deep end and invest in a lifetime supply of chocolate bars, just keep in mind that a healthier choice is raw cacao or carob powder - both have even higher levels of magnesium which is ultimately what your body needs. So go ahead…indulge in these better choices! Choose dark chocolate that is over 80 percent cocoa and skip the guilt of the sugar laden milk chocolate. Or, try other foods that are high in magnesium like celery and sunflower seeds. You may also consider a consider a magnesium supplement to kick those cravings to the curb before they take over your life!

Ingredients

- ½ cup almonds
- ½ cup walnuts
- 1 cup dates (pitted)
- handful sunflower seeds
- 2 tbsp carob powder
- 2 tbsp hemp seeds
- 1 tsp vanilla
- sea salt to taste
- 2 tsp sea veggie powder (can be found at the health food store) or greens powder
- optional – sprinkle of dark chocolate chips
- optional – roll in unsweetened coconut

Directions

Blend nuts in food processor until finely ground almost to a powder. Add dates, carob powder, sunflower seeds, hemp seeds, vanilla and sea veggie powder and blend. Mixture should be slightly moist so that you can roll them into balls. Roll in coconut if desired.

DID YOU KNOW?

Raw food is loaded with natural enzymes, important in the metabolism of foods. Unfortunately, cooking or processing destroys the natural enzymes which means your body has to draw on its own store of enzymes to assist in the breakdown of foods - which takes energy! Enzymes are an important key to improved nutrient absorption and vibrant health.

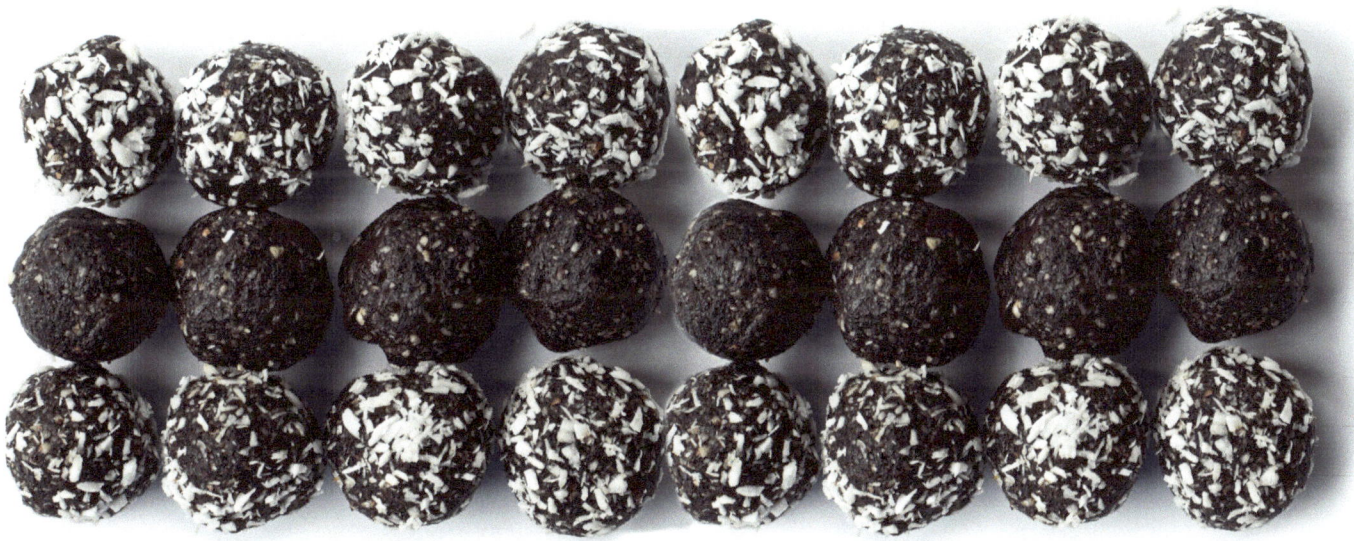

nutritional nibble...

You might be picturing a tree hugging, long haired hippy after reading the word hemp. Ahem…we don't mean that kind of hemp. Hemp seeds, otherwise known as cannabis sativa, (no we don't mean that kind of cannabis…) are just seeds that contain all the essential amino acids and essential fatty acids necessary to maintain healthy human life in the most easily digested form. Wow! So go ahead and get a natural energy high! You can use hemp seeds on salads, in soups, or in plain yogurt for that extra crunch and nutrition. Sea greens are rich in both potassium and iodine making them an excellent choice for thyroid balance. If your thyroid does not have enough iodine, then insufficient thyroxine is produced and too much estrogen builds up. This puts strain on the liver and fatigue, anger and even weight gain may result.

Black Bean Spirulina Brownie: Makes 12 brownies

You might have PMS if a sword fight for the last brownie doesn't seem like a ridiculous idea at all. Hopefully you've been using the anti-PMS recipes and your cravings have lessened. But cravings will happen. And like a good soldier ready to do battle, you don't want to fight the war unarmed. Okay, a little dramatic, but let's just say it doesn't hurt to have an awesome, healthy brownie recipe in your arsenal for when that craving hits. So here you go…consider yourself armed.

Ingredients

- 1 can black beans, drained and rinsed
- 3 hormone-free eggs
- ½ cup sucanat sugar (or 1/3 cup agave nectar)
- ½ cup cocoa powder
- ¼ cup pumpkin
- 2 tbsp coconut oil, melted
- 2 tsp vanilla
- 1 tbsp spirulina powder (optional)
- ½ cup dark chocolate chips (over 70 percent) or chop up a dark chocolate bar
- Optional – food grade peppermint oil or 1 tsp coffee

Directions

Preheat oven to 375°F. Blend beans, eggs, sugar, cocoa, oil, vanilla and spirulina until smooth. Grease an 8 x 8 inch pan with coconut oil and then coat with cocoa powder to prevent sticking. Pour brownie mixture into pan and then sprinkle chocolate chips on top. Use a knife to mix them in slightly, leaving a few on top. Bake for 30 minutes or until the top feels firm to touch.

DID YOU KNOW?

If you eat as many superfoods, like spirulina, as possible prior to the onset of your period, this will not only ensure that you are nutritionally balanced but it will help decrease any symptoms you typically experience. Other super foods to try are; wild blue-green algae, maca powder, chlorella, and royal jelly.

nutritional nibble…

Spirulina is a cultivated micro algae, with one of the richest levels of protein found in a natural food. It contains 60 – 70% protein while meat contains only about 25% complete protein. It also contains vital minerals such as iron, vitamins B12, RNA and DNA and essential fatty acids. Spirulina can help control blood sugar and associated cravings so it is a great food for those wishing to lose weight. If that's not a good excuse to eat a chocolate brownie, we don't know what is!

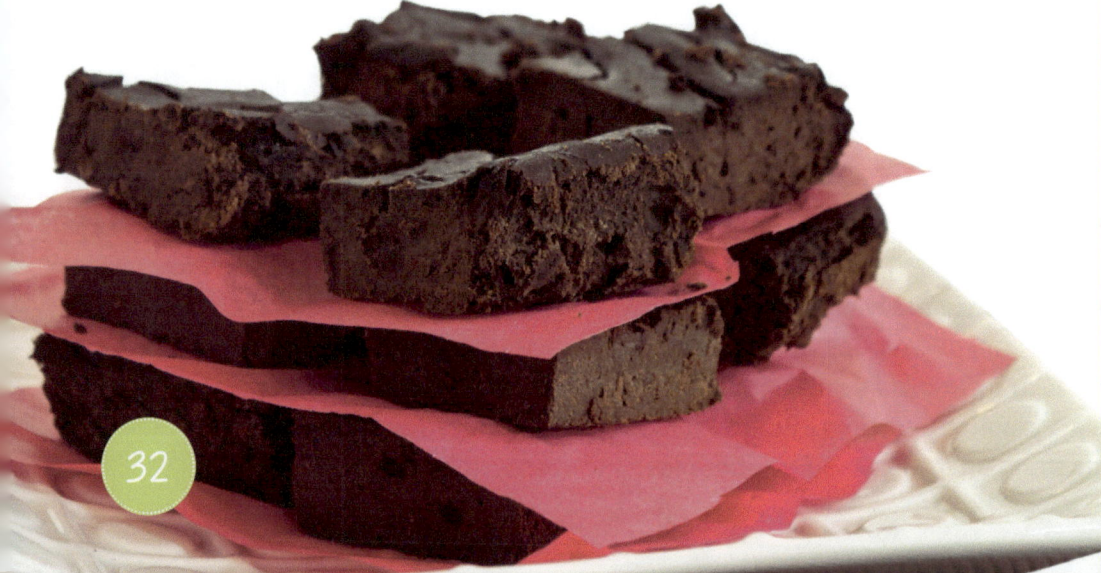

Here is yet another weapon for your craving arsenal. A super food version of the standard Reese peanut butter cups. WARNING: These are addictive!

Ingredients

- ⅓ cup peanut butter (or almond butter)
- 1 date with a sprinkle of unsweetened coconut
- 1 tbsp ground flax seeds or hemp seeds
- 3 tbsp water
- 1 tsp pure vanilla extract
- pinch sea salt
- ½ cup cacao powder
- ½ cup coconut oil
- 2 tsp maca powder
- 1 tsp agave or honey or stevia (or to taste)

NUTRITIONAL NIBBLE

Dates are a wonderful way to sweeten up your desserts. Dates won't raise blood sugars as quickly as refined sugars, especially when mixed with a healthy fat and fibre. They are also an excellent whole food perfect for increasing energy levels. However, be careful that you don't overdo them because they are one of the higher GI fruits out there.

Directions

Blend peanut butter, coconut, dates, ground flax seeds or hemp seeds, vanilla and sea salt in a food processor until smooth. Melt coconut oil and cacao powder in a small pot on very low heat until melted. Add maca powder and agave. Pour a little of the melted chocolate into small paper lined cups, coating the sides lightly by pushing the chocolate up the sides. Pop into the freezer to set. Remove when set and then put a teaspoon of peanut butter mixture into each cup and then coat with remaining chocolate. Put into the freezer until set.

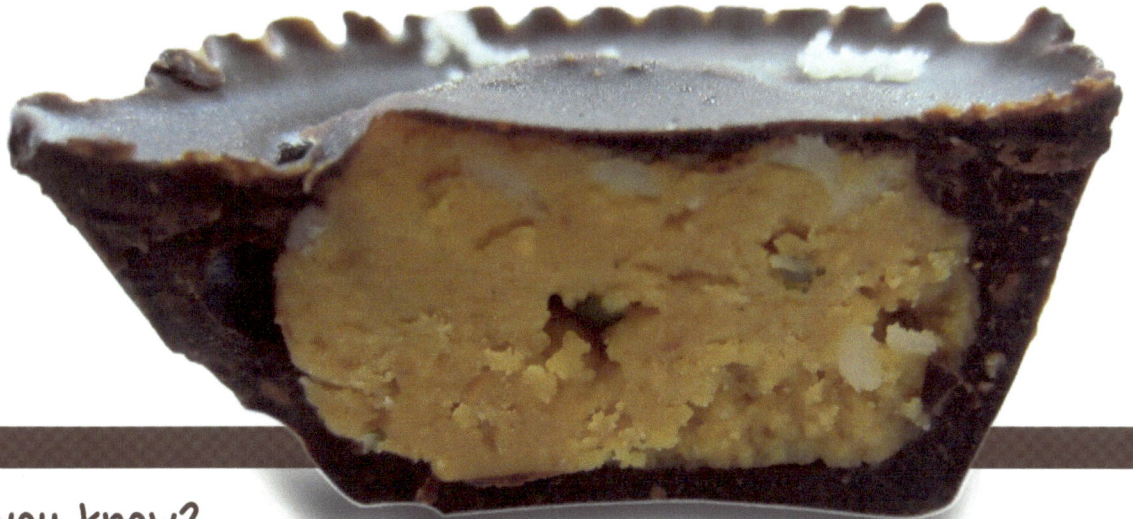

Did you know?

Most of us know that nuts and seeds are vital for their healthy fats and protein ratio but did you know that they are also important for their Vitamin E content? Studies show a reduction in the symptoms of PMS by increasing Vitamin E. A handful of nuts a day will do, just make sure the nuts and seeds are raw and not the roasted variety which are typically loaded with salt and rancid oils that burden your liver. Remember you need a healthy liver to help reduce PMS.

Raw Key Lime Pie: Serves 10 - 12

Its tough getting all of the nutrition we need in just 3 meals a day, so we made sure we put nutrition into our desserts as well. This is a delicious guilt free dessert option, filled with fibre, healthy fats and ingredients that will help fight PMS. This is a fun way to eat avocado and you won't even know it's there.

Ingredients

Crust

- 1 ½ cups oats
- ½ cup coconut
- 1 tbsp flax seeds, ground
- 6 medjool dates
- 1 tbsp melted coconut oil
- pinch sea salt

Filling

- 2 avocados
- juice from 3 limes
- lime zest from one lime
- 1 tsp vanilla extract
- ¼ cup agave nectar or sweetener of choice
- 1 can coconut milk (put in fridge for a couple hours and then use only the thick milk from top of can)
- ½ cup powdered sugar (you could skip this if you don't mind things less sweet)

RECIPE TIP

Make sure the avocados you select are not too firm. You want them to be soft enough to blend into a creamy texture.

Directions

Grease a 9 inch spring form pan and then set aside. Put oats and coconut into food processor and blend until fine. Add sea salt. Remove pits from dates and then add to mixture along with coconut oil and blend again. Mixture should hold together when you press it together. Press crust into 9 inch spring form pan and put in fridge.

Blend avocados, lime juice, lime rind, agave nectar and vanilla. Remove coconut milk from fridge and then scoop the thick part off the top and put in separate bowl. Add powdered sugar and then blend well until thick. Fold coconut mixture into lime mixture and then pour into crust. Place in freezer and remove about 20 minutes before serving.

nutritional nibble...

Adding ground flax seeds or chia seeds to your meals throughout the day will support your digestive system by providing fibre which will help keep things moving along. The basis of good health is a well-functioning digestive system. You don't want your body to eliminate your food so fast that you don't absorb nutrition or so slow that your body can't get rid of toxins quickly enough.

Nothing says Autumn like Pumpkin. Pumpkin pie, pumpkin muffins, pumpkin spiced lattes; our taste buds are tempted by the wonderful aroma and taste of pumpkin! Now, it can feel like fall all year round with this recipe. Try this version of a latte that will entice your palette with all the flavours of Fall without all the PMS aggravating sugar and caffeine. We think it's the perfect afternoon pick me up. Don't worry, with this recipe you won't have to sacrifice your health or aggravate your PMS because this is a caffeine and sugar-free pick me up.

Ingredients

- 1 cup of strongly brewed teeccino or any natural 'coffee-free' coffee (1 tbsp per cup)
- 1 cup of full fat, unsweetened coconut milk
- 1 cup of water or almond milk
- 4 tbsp pumpkin puree
- ¼ tsp ground cinnamon
- pinch of both ground nutmeg and cloves
- 2 – 4 tbsp honey, stevia or coconut sugar
- ½ tsp vanilla

Directions

Make the teeccino as per package directions. Place the milk, pumpkin, spices, and honey into a small pot and bring to a simmer. Add the teeccino and the vanilla. Adjust with more sweetener or spices, if desired. Pour into two large mugs and share with someone you love.

Did you know?

A grande pumpkin spice latte has 49 g of sugar, or 12.25 tsp. Yikes! That is definitely NOT low glycemic. But don't worry, you can still get that 'sweet' taste you crave without adding refined sugar and impacting your insulin levels negatively. There are a variety of sugars available now that are considered low glycemic. Keep it low with stevia, agave nectar, coconut nectar, yacon syrup, Xylitol, or erythritol. Be careful to introduce xylitol or erythritol into your diet slowly because it has been found to cause digestive issues for some. The best most natural choice is stevia with coconut sugar as our runner up.

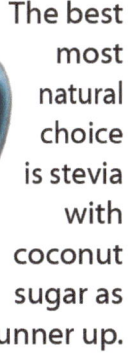

How to put it all together:

Phew! You made it through another month. But what about next month? Sometimes it just takes a little planning. Start now and you should feel better for your next cycle. For those of you who are too busy or overwhelmed to make your own menu plan with these recipes, we have provided a sample menu plan below for 5 days of PMS symptom free eating. Give it a try, and see what happens! Feel free to mix and match all snacks and meals. It's more important to look at your diet nutritionally over the week than it is to look at it over one day. If you don't get many veggies on one day, no biggie, just eat more the next day and your body will do its thing to keep you going.

Sample Menu Plan for PMS Prevention

	Day 1	Day 2	Day 3	Day 4	Day 5
Breakfast	PMS Oatmeal or Protein shake	2 poached eggs with 1 slice sprouted rye bread, smothered in coconut oil & mashed avocado	Protein Shake with greens powder or PMS Oatmeal	2 egg veggie omelette with goat cheese feta	Protein pancakes with fresh fruit topping and Greek yogurt sweetened with stevia
Snack	Handful seeds (pumpkin, sunflower) or greens drink	2 raw Omega balls or green drink	Handful raw almonds or green drink	Against the Grain Banana and Walnut Muffin	Sliced apple dipped in 1 tbsp nut butter or green drink
Lunch	Romaine salad with chopped chicken & avocado Optional whole grain crackers	Turkey Lasagna & broccoli slaw salad	Salt and Pepper Shrimp Salad & sprouted grain bread	Lentil Chia Soup Whole grain tortilla – toasted	Shrimp Napa Cabbage Salad or leftover tuna pasta
Snack	Apple with 1 tbsp nut butter	Veggies with hummus	Guacamole with whole grain crackers or a boiled egg	Black Bean Brownie or veggies and nut butter	Hummus with veggies
Dinner	Turkey Lasagna & Spinach Salad	Shrimp and veggie stir fry with brown rice or Skinny Meatloaf	Almond Crusted Halibut with steamed kale	Tuna pasta with Avocado Salad	Burritos with steamed greens
Optional Snack	Celery and tahini or Pumpkin Latte	Warm unsweetened almond milk	Raw Cacao Pudding or cucumber with goat cheese	1 slice whole grain toast with nut butter	1 cup Coconut Oil Popcorn or any snack

Feel free to eat any of the following snacks as they are all low GI and are focused on PMS prevention:

- Handful seeds (pumpkin, sunflower)
- Handful nuts (raw almonds, raw walnuts, etc)
- Celery with nut butter and raisins
- Cucumber and goat cheese
- Popcorn popped in coconut oil and seasoned with sea salt
- Almond milk
- Veggies and hummus
- Raw Power Balls
- Protein shake
- Veggies and nut butter
- Whole grain tortilla with hummus
- Guacamole with veggies and/or rice crackers
- Brown Rice Cake with nut butter and ground flax
- Hard-boiled egg (free run and hormone free)
- Herbal tea (optional, mix in 1 tbsp. ground flax seeds)

In moderation:

- 1 oz dark chocolate (over 80 percent is best)
- Full fat Greek style yogurt sprinkled with seeds and stevia and/or cocoa powder
- Whole grain muffins

References

Bowden, Jonny, PhD. C.N.S., *The Healthiest Meals on Earth.*
Fair Winds Press, MA, 2008

Colbin, AnneMarie, *Food and Healing.*
The Random House Ballantine Publishing Group, NY, 1986.

David, William, M.D. *Wheat Belly.*
HarperCollins Publishers Ltd., Ontario, 2012

Dupont, Caroline Marie, *Enlightened Eating.*
Books Alive, TN, 2006

Haas, Elson, M.D., *Staying Healthy with Nutrition.*
Celestial Arts Publishing, California, 1992

Tart-Jensen, Ellen, *Health is Your Birthright.*
Celestial Arts, California, 2006

Wright, Jonathan, M.D., *Library of Food and Vitamin Cures.*
Newmarket Health Publishing, Maryland, 2011

Websites:
http://www.balancepointhc.com/blog/
http://www.canadianliving.com
http://www.chatelaine.com
http://www.doh.wa.gov/ehp/oehas/fish/fishchart. html

Many recipes were inspired by those found on **chatelaine.com** and **canadianliving.com**.